The 5:2 Diet

Intermittent Fasting to Lose Weight and Better Health

By Shawn Reath

Introduction

I want to thank you and congratulate you for downloading the book, *"The 5:2 Diet: Intermittent Fasting to Lose Weight and Better Health."*

This book contains proven steps and strategies on how to lose weight and gain better health through intermittent fasting especially the 5:2 diet. This book will explain why intermittent fasting is better than going on a diet. It is also going to show you how easy it is to do intermittent fasting through the 5:2 diet as compared to other methods.

If diets compel you to eat certain foods and to avoid others, then intermittent fasting might just be what you are looking for. If you are wary of eating particular foods or you don't want a regimen of physical activity, then you might enjoy the low impact of intermittent fasting. If you are scared that you might turn to binge eating or become dizzy, light-headed, or unable to cope with hunger spells, have no fear. The 5:2 diet or intermittent fasting plan will ensure you won't run out of energy or end up in the hospital. It is guaranteed to take into account all that you are capable of without imposing health risks.

Be assured, intermittent fasting has no adverse side effects. It is easier on your body than Paleo or any other diet and you won't have to cut out any of your favorite foods. And the best thing about it is you are guaranteed weight loss and better health.

Thanks again for downloading this book, I hope you enjoy it!

Why You Should Read This Book

This book will help you finally discover the best solution to better health and weight loss. That is one good reason to read this book. Another good reason to read this book is to know why intermittent fasting is so much better that dieting.

If you have been disappointed by the insignificant results of dieting or its imposition and restrictions, it's time to consider intermittent fasting. Intermittent fasting doesn't have food restrictions, portion control or calorie limits. Read and find out how this is possible. And while you're at it, read how intermittent fasting can get you the results you want faster and with less stress on your body or your appetite.

Finally, if you still think that intermittent fasting is not for you, read this book to discover how losing weight and being healthy does not require something bland, restrictive, or complicated. This book just might have what you need to be able to enjoy good meals, your favorite food, and some guaranteed and effective way of getting the weight that you want and achieve the level of health you crave.

Copyright

Disclaimer

The information provided in this book is designed to provide helpful information on the subjects discussed. This book is not meant to be used, nor should it be used, to diagnose or treat any medical condition. For diagnosis or treatment of any medical problem, consult your own physician. The publisher and author are not responsible for any specific health or allergy needs that may require medical supervision and are not liable for any damages or negative consequences from any treatment, action, application or preparation, to any person reading or following the information in this book. Any references included are provided for informational purposes only and do not constitute endorsement of any websites or other sources. Readers should be aware that any websites listed in this book may change.

Why You Should Read This Book

This book will help you finally discover the best solution to better health and weight loss. That is one good reason to read this book. Another good reason to read this book is to know why intermittent fasting is so much better that dieting.

If you have been disappointed by the insignificant results of dieting or its imposition and restrictions, it's time to consider intermittent fasting. Intermittent fasting doesn't have food restrictions, portion control or calorie limits. Read and find out how this is possible. And while you're at it, read how intermittent fasting can get you the results you want faster and with less stress on your body or your appetite.

Finally, if you still think that intermittent fasting is not for you, read this book to discover how losing weight and being healthy does not require something bland, restrictive, or complicated. This book just might have what you need to be able to enjoy good meals, your favorite food, and some guaranteed and effective way of getting the weight that you want and achieve the level of health you crave.

Copyright

Disclaimer

Table of Contents

Diet vs. Intermittent Fasting

In the search for better health and weight loss, people have been on the lookout for a more effective diet. Finally there is one that is going to give all other diets such as vegan, Paleo, South Beach, and any other celebrity-endorsed diet a run for their money. No, it's not another diet. It's a lifestyle change that many have been practicing for thousands of years. It's intermittent fasting.

Proponents of diet have long held sway over the fitness world with promises of improved health and weight loss. Unfortunately that promise has been short-lived and the word "diet" has come to mean something that is unsustainable and bound to fail after sometime. On the other hand, fasting as a measure of health and religious significance has been practiced since the dawn of time when humans didn't always have food readily available and therefore needed to master their appetites.

Even today, intermittent fasting or fasting in general has several advantages over dieting:

Less Food restriction

The critical component of a diet's success is its reduction of calories. In a typical diet, that means not eating certain kinds of food such as grains, beans, or bread for Paleo, meat and fish for vegan, and certain foods for Mediterranean and South Beach. These diets claim the avoidance is necessary not only to provide the necessary calorie reduction but also to reduce the intake of antinutrients and empty calories that do not contribute to good health. Unfortunately, these mean less interesting, bland, and generally depressing foods to eat. That is the primary reason why most diets fail. It's not because the diet doesn't work but the food restriction leaves the dieter too deprived to enjoy eating.

With intermittent fasting, the type of food doesn't matter as much as the quantity cut. Some fasting methods don't impose a ban on processed foods, sodas or animal fat. It only asked that you either stop eating or reduce the normal intake of food during fasting periods. This makes it more tolerable for people to skip meals or eat a reduced portion.

Less Complex to Follow

With the food restrictions that some diets impose come the need to go out of your way to shop and prepare for unfamiliar and less savory meals like green smoothies, salads, non-whole grain bread, etc. It also cuts deep into your wallet as you go off in search of organic, natural, and free-range poultry. These types of food are usually not readily accessible and generally more expensive. Thus, even though a diet is satisfying and looks very promising, sustaining it may not be feasible.

With intermittent fasting, the restriction on food does not go beyond the "eat less of" directive. Off course, it is in anyone's best interest to eat a balanced meal and that is the same thing that intermittent fasting asks. It does not however require you to break the bank in order to achieve weight loss and better health.

Restores Fat as the Body's Primary Fuel Source

Diets attempt to restore fat as the body's primary source of fuel. However if your diet continues to have starch, carbohydrates and sugar, your body will keep burning that for energy. And if your diet includes gluten-rich food like bread and processed food like hotdogs, your body ends up with undesirable by-products like free radicals.

Research shows that intermittent fasting restores fat as the body's primary fuel. Through a process called ketosis, the deprivation of carbohydrates to burn from the absence of food forces your body to use fat for fuel. Intermittent fasting also causes the regular secretion of HGH, a hormone that utilizes the body's fat cells to produce energy.

With intermittent fasting, your body adapts a cycle of ketosis to keep metabolizing your body's fat for energy. This reduces the layer of fatty deposits and as long as you do not reintroduce high levels of sugar or carbohydrates through binge eating, your body will continue to burn fat.

Reduces Sugar Dependence

Diets have a hard time breaking the sugar dependence especially if your diet is so restrictive. However, with intermittent fasting, your body gets used to regularly burn fat instead of sugar, thus making you less dependent on the latter. This actually programs your body to crave less for sweets and lose the appetite for sugary foods. That is good news for your body as the risk of acute and chronic diseases like diabetes, hypertension and cardiovascular disease is greatly reduced.

Reduces Insulin and Leptin Resistance

Vegan diets and other diets high in antioxidant food attempt to overcome insulin resistance which happens as a result of eating too much sugar-rich and processed food. However even a diet of fruit and vegetables has sugar levels that can slow down the reduction of insulin resistance and cause the body's cells to leak fat, amino acids and glucose. It also causes your body to increase the size of its fat cells through leptin resistance.

Trough intermittent fasting, your body forces the secretion of leptin to normalize the sensitivity of the cells in your body to insulin. This boosts the ability of your body's cells to produce mitochondrial energy and metabolize fat. The result is a reduction of insulin and leptin resistance which in turn makes your body burn your fat cells for energy rather than increase in size.

Controls and Reduces Craving and Appetite

The ancients have long used fasting as a means to discipline the body's passions, desires, and appetites. On the other hand, diet attempts to curb that by reducing sugar dependence and replacing the craving for something else. This is because eating sugar-rich food including carbs and starches inhibits the normal function of a hormone known as ghrelin. Ghrelin controls your craving and balances your body's weight and energy levels. Ghrelin levels rise when your weight drops and triggers craving then fall when you gain it back in order to make you lose appetite. Sugar suppresses that and diets do little to control ghrelin levels. However, intermittent fasting normalizes ghrelin levels allowing them to rise and fall normally and burn fat through metabolism. This regulates your cravings and appetite.

Detoxifies

Dieting has been said to detoxify the body through the introduction of antioxidant-rich food. However, the body already has its own detoxifying process called autophagy. This is how the body naturally cleanses and replaces worn out parts of the mitochondrial parts of the body's cells. There are however wastes called AGE or advanced glycation end-products that accumulate in cellular tissues and cannot be dislodged. Unless removed, AGE leads to plaque build-up in arteries and veins causing stroke. Through intermittent fasting, however, the body can trigger a process called ketosis which burns away these wastes along with the body's fat cells.

Weight Loss and Better Health

Given the benefits and advantages of intermittent fasting over dieting, the combined effect of using up fat, normalizing insulin, leptin and ghrelin levels and reducing sugar dependence, cravings and appetites, one can seriously expect better health and a resulting weight loss. With the added benefit of detoxification, intermittent fasting has distinct advantages over dieting especially when it removes the severe food restrictions that make it difficult for dieters to maintain a diet.

Should it be any wonder then why you shouldn't choose to do intermittent fasting rather than dieting?

What is 5:2 Intermittent Fasting?

Having learned why intermittent fasting is a much better option than dieting, the question now goes down to what would be the best option for weight loss and better health?

With so many methods for intermittent fasting available, it can be difficult to choose. There are intermittent fasting methods that only ask you to fast for a 24 period and others which ask you to do so part of the day. How effective they are in losing weight and giving you better health will be discussed in the next chapter. This book however recommends an intermittent fasting method that is easy on most individuals and does not strain beginners. It was also one of the first fasting for health techniques and popularized by the book, *The Fast Diet: Lose Weight, Stay Healthy, and Live Longer with the Simple Secret of Intermittent Fasting* by Dr. Michael Mosley.

This method is the 5:2 Diet, The Fast Diet, or the 5:2 Intermittent Fasting plan.

The 5:2 intermittent fasting is very easy. All it requires you to do is pick two days in a week for fasting and use the remaining five days to eat normally. Proponents of intermittent fasting prefer to call these days "Feast" days and "Fast" days.

Fast Days

The 5:2 diet is named such because it stands for five days of "feast" or days when you eat normally and two "fast" days where your food intake is below normal. The term diet is actually a misnomer because there are no prescribed food although the expectation is for you to eat healthy and normally.

So what do you do on Fast days?

Dr. Michael Mosley and his followers have a few recommendations:

1. **Pick your Two Days**

    Your Fast days can start on a Monday followed by three days eating normally. Your next fast day can then be Friday. Some recommend Tuesday and Friday for your fast days.

    Dr. Mosley and most proponents of the 5:2 Diet recommend that you begin fasting on a day where you are nominally busy so that you have something to keep your mind of food. A suggestion will be to have breakfast on Monday and then start your fast beginning at lunch and then break it at lunch or dinner time on Tuesday. If you are beginning, then it is alright for you to break it at breakfast on a Tuesday. A similar schedule can be done starting your fast on lunch Friday and breaking it Saturday at breakfast or lunch. You might want to avoid running into Friday night dinners by scheduling you fast to start on Thursday and end on Friday.

Keep your fasting schedule fixed so that your body can program your metabolism and make the necessary adjustments to adapt to this fasting schedule.

2. Eat Less

So does your fasting have to involve total abstinence from food and water? Certainly not! Dr. Mosley instead recommends eating foods that are the most satiating even if these are in one fourth of the amounts that you would have normally. That is the basic principle of this plan or diet. Some of these foods could be meat, fish or even vegetables so long as they are high in protein and fiber.

From a calorie perspective, your food intake during the entire period of your fast should be as low as 400-500 calories for the entire fasting period. This means you can have a smoothie or a protein shake that you can sip throughout the day if that makes it easier for you to get adjusted to your fast. However, having one small meal during the day is actually netter than having several mini-meals or snacks.

3. Drink More

Yes. You can drink water or any zero-calorie drinks during your fast days.

"Feast" Days

Dr. Mosley recommends eating a well balance meal during your "feast" or normal days. He does not suggest any foods to avoid or stay away from much less eat less of. He and his proponents suggest making no changes to the amount or the kind of food that you normally eat nor does he recommend changing your meal schedule.

The one thing that Dr. Mosley warns beginners or anyone trying out the 5:2 diet is to avoid binge eating particularly before your fast or just after it. What this does is it actually messes up any gains you've made during days that you fasted and disrupts your metabolism. To avoid binge eating you can use any calorie counter programs to measure your food intake before and after fasting. Keeping it at 2000 to 2,500 calories is a good idea. You can also plan your meals ahead of time and home-cook them so you won't be tempted to eat out and order everything on the menu.

As you start doing this, the 5:2 diet is guaranteed to give you the results you have been waiting to have even better health and guaranteed weight loss.

Advantages of 5:2 over Other IF Variants

As mentioned, there are various forms of intermittent fasting. So why pick 5:2 instead of any of the others?

To understand, here's a look at what the other forms are so you can make the right choice:

Eat-Stop-Eat

This form of intermittent fasting was popularized by Brad Pilon, a leading expert and author if *Eat Stop Eat*. His method is very similar to 5:2 except for one thing: instead of a reduced meal during fast days, he suggests you have nothing but water for a 24 hour period. It's that simple. And it doesn't have to be 2 days just as long as the fasting period is a straight 24 hours. The rest of the days, feel free to eat normally.

The benefits are the same as 5:2. However, this type of intermittent fasting finds that 24 hours without food is long enough to give them symptoms of light-headedness, dizziness, hunger, or even fatigue. While Pilon explains that his method is flexible enough to allow people to start small until they are able to completely fast, most people cant. It also imposes a bit of trouble when social events such as dinners occur during a fasting period.

Pilon's method allows your body to get into ketosis quickly and thereby hasten weight loss if you are able to bear the 24 hour fast. However, the absence of food can tempt you to snack or binge-eat after the fast which can throw away your gains during the fasting period. However, this method has one advantage over 5:2 and that it removes the need to count calories or measure portions during the fasting periods.

Leangain

This method was developed by Martain Beckhan for people who like to work out in the gym. It's a very fast way to lose weight and get trim especially for folks who combine weight training with fasting.

This method is different from 5:2 and Eat-Stop-Eat in that it takes the day instead of the week and divides it into "fasting" and "feeding" times. "Fasting" time is a period including sleep where no food consumption is allowed. You could however drink water, zero-calorie soda, sugarless tea or coffee and any other calorie-free drinks. You can also chew sugarless and calorie-free gum. Fasting time is about 16 hours for men and 14 hours for women.

"Feeding" time is a 5-10 hour window where meals are allowed. This usually starts some 4-6 hours after waking up. During this time, you can have as many as three meals. Just make sure that the feeding window remains consistent in order not to mess up any gains you made while fasting.

In addition to watching out for feeding time, LeanGains requires that you match each day with workouts and let that determine what you are having during the day's feeding time. For instance, if you are not working out, eat fat and when you are, eat carb-rich food. That also means making sure you get sufficient protein based on your workout goals.

Leangains is an intermittent fasting method that is guaranteed to make you trim but is a tough regimen to follow for non-body building types. If you are simply trying to lose weight and gain better health, you are better off leaving this method to the more athletic types.

Warrior's Diet

The Warrior's Diet is a variation of LeanGains rather than 5:2 or Eat-Stop-Eat which means you might want to stay away from trying out this method unless having one meal a night appeals to you. With the Warrior's Diet, you extend the fasting period to as much as 20 hours and the feeding period to only a few hours at night. That should be just sufficient for a single large meal that is packed with proteins, carbohydrates and all the necessary nutrients.

This idea of a eating a large meal at night is to make sure your body gets in sync with your circadian cycle and take advantage of the Parasympathetic Nervous System to calm, digest and relax your body.

On the other hand, the fasting period allows you to drink water or fresh juice or eat a small serving of vegetables, fruit, fish, or meat in order to stimulate the burning of fat and the release of energy.

Again, this is a much regimented fasting method that can hinder you if you are not used to eating once a day and at night at that. However, military types, athletes, body builders and serious weight watchers prefer the Warrior's Diet because it can really speed up fat loss. It is certainly not for anyone with regular day job.

Alternate Day Fasting

Finally, if you want to speed up weight loss but you do not want the extremes of LeanGains and Warrior's or the no-food requirement of Eat-Stop-Eat, alternate fasting is the next step after 5:2. Here you simply replicate your fast and feast days and make it every other day. Just like the 5:2, you drop your fast day consumption to about a fourth or a fifth of what you normally have. You can choose to have one single midday meal during fast days or eat a series of mini meals or smoothies just like with 5:2.

Again, the danger here is to binge eat so carefully planning your meals is very important. This way, your metabolism continues to burn fat as fuel and your insulin, leptin and ghrelin levels remain regulated and normal.

Alternate day fasting is a natural progression of 5:2 and can be a stepping stone to Eat-Stop-Eat in order to lose weight and gain better health.

Benefits of 5:2 Intermittent Fasting

So is the 5:2 Diet or method of intermittent fasting for you? In order to better understand if it is, examine the following benefits:

5:2 offers a manageable schedule of fasting

Intermittent fasting employs fasting by schedules. From the comparisons done on the other methods, 5:2 would have the simplest and most manageable schedule. A person shifting from a normal non-fasting daily schedule will not be stymied by a 14-36 fasting hour period that can be stressful. On the other hand, the two full days of fasting that comes with 6:2 will not be too difficult to follow especially since the person is still allowed a small meal. This means that metabolism, insulin, leptin, and ghrelin levels will not go awry or experience a drastic change. The extremes of a single large meal or a daily longer period for fasting which usually breaks the back of anyone who wants to try out intermittent fasting will not be encountered.

Manageable Weight Loss

The 5:2 intermittent fasting method is a wonderful way to lose weight. The drop in 23 days out of 5 is sufficient to stimulate fat burning that will have the net effect losing two to two and a half pounds a week. In fact Dr. Michael Mosley, proponent of the 5:2 diet has revealed that he has lost 19 pounds in just 2 months of following the 5:2 intermittent fasting method. This is because intermittent fasting forces the body to go through a metabolic cycle that feeds off its fat reserves. Fasting triggers ketosis which in turn causes fat burning. Additional hormonal releases such as HGH trigger further fat utilization.

Dr. Mosley's experience confirms the findings of studies as early as 1939 when scientists started researching the benefits of fasting. Their findings from cultural observations on non-religious fasting indicated that a longer duration between meals actually produce better health and weight loss than dieting, They specifically discovered that individuals who fasted twice a week then ate whatever they wanted for the remaining period had lesser risks to health and faster fat loss.

Lifestyle Change

Unlike diets which are essentially meal plans and lists of what to eat or avoid, intermittent fasting is a lifestyle change that requires you to modify eating schedules and skipping or reducing the amount of food eaten. This requires if necessary a change in schedule to ensure that activities are not affected by the switch to fasting such as weekend dinners, bar hopping, or dining out. It also necessitates an additional change in activities such as exercise, physical activities and working from home.

The lifestyle changes allow you to cope up with the initial symptoms of fasting until it becomes easy to follow. The 5:2 intermittent fasting method makes it even easier to do as it has less of the symptoms of diet change like cravings, flatulence, irritability, light-headedness or hunger pangs. It also does not automatically lead to binge eating. In fact, most adherents of 5:2 rarely fall into binge eating and their energy levels remain constant whether they fast or not.

Better Health

Even though intermittent fasting recommends a reduction of total calories consumed rather than a ban on certain food, it still results into better health. This is because of the following:

Disease Prevention

Because intermittent fasting normalizes insulin, ghrelin, and leptin levels, it causes the body to decrease oxidative stress and chronic excessive inflammation which in turn cause free radical accumulation and cell and tissue damage. This suppresses the risk of debilitating diseases like hypertension, diabetes and even cancer.

5:2 intermittent fasting can regularly lower triglycerides levels by metabolizing fat cells which lowers the risk of contracting stroke, hypertension, obesity and diabetes. It also improves insulin sensitivity which improves your blood sugar levels and with it your risk of avoiding diabetes or cardiovascular diseases.

Statistical analysis of the effects of intermittent fasting indicates that it decreases the risk of food-related diseases by as much as 30 percent with a corresponding increase in longevity.

Improves Mental Health

Scientific studies on intermittent fasting identified that the production of ketones when the body starts metabolizing fat enables new growth of mitochondria and an increase of glutathione in the hippocampus of the brain protecting it from infection and inflammation. This makes fasting a potential tool in the treatment of dementia, depression and even Parkinson's. Ketones can also grow new neural pathways making fasting another potential tool for the treatment of Alzheimer's.

Fasting also produces brain-derived neurotropic factor or BDNF which converts the brain's stem cells into new neurons which protect the brain from cellular changes due to Alzheimer's, Huntington's and Parkinson's diseases. According to the National Institute on Aging simple fasting or reduces one's consumption to 600 calories every other day can increase BDNF levels by as much as 400 percent.

Anti-aging

When intermittent fasting stimulates the secretion of HGH or the human growth hormone, it metabolizes fat, promotes muscle repair and growth and tightens the skin. This anti-aging effect makes people feel and look younger than they really are. Indeed, research has shown that fasting intermittently, boosts HGH production in women by 1400 percent and in men by 2000. This results into faster recovery from muscle fatigue, greater physical endurance and automatic skin tightening which produces a slender, younger looking physique.

The 5:2 intermittent fasting method can decrease free radical production by preventing further damage to cell proteins, nucleic acids and lipids due to oxidative stress and the aging process. Finally, it also normalizes insulin sensitivity and inhibits the mTOR pathway to slow down aging, resulting in a more youthful glow.

5:2 Intermittent Fasting FAQ's

Before you try out the 5:2 Diet or intermittent fasting method, here are a few FAQ's to keep in mind:

Can you begin fasting after dinner?

Fasting can be done by anyone and there is nothing wrong to start your fast after dinner. This will just make fasting easier because it takes advantage of sleep and your circadian rhythm to metabolize and allow cellular detoxification to take place.

When should I fast?

Fast at a time when your mind is busy and you are too preoccupied to think about eating. This means don't begin fasting when you are relaxing on a weekend. Chances are the lack of food and activity will force you to want to eat more than you are allowed to.

That said, don't schedule fast days on a weekend, holiday, or for that matter on Friday dinners, Monday brunches, or social events. You should either have a good excuse to miss these activities or revise your schedule.

Can I Exercise?

You certainly can perform regular exercise during your fast days. Evidence suggests that there is no risk to health when you do. Just do not engage in serious weight training or hard core work outs. Here are a couple of guidelines to remember in order to make exercise work:

> **Perform low-intensity cardio when fasting**
> When fasting, limit exercises to low-intensity cardio routines such as a brisk walk or a light jog. These are sufficient exercises and should not get you into trouble. You can do upper body exercises, squats, splits, pushups but make sure you are able to carry out a conversation in mid-exercising. Pay close attention to how you feel and stop exercising if you start to run short of breath, feel light-headed or dizzy. Don't increase the intensity or it could do you more harm than good. Low intensity cardio should be sufficient to jumpstart your metabolism.

> Drink water to keep hydrated during your work out.

> **Do high-intensity workouts after you have eaten.**
> Maximize fat loss while having lots of energy by scheduling your workouts as close to your last meal. Feel free to have workout sessions of moderate to high intensity including weight training. This will ensure you have sufficient glycogen to burn as you workout.

Have a carb-rich snack to replenish your body's depleted fuel sources after you complete any high-intensity workout to avoid switching from burning fat to burning glycogen. Make sure you eat protein-rich food before and after your workouts as well and that you are well-nourished before starting another fasting session. Never do intermittent fasting unless your workouts are well within your feast days. Sandwich them between two snacks, a snack and a meal or two meals and always make sure to load up on carbs and protein.

Can I have a snack while fasting?

Take advantage of the flexibility that intermittent fasting allows with regard to eating snacks and meals. Consuming a snack or a meal 3 -4 hours before you hit the gym ensures that you will have enough energy to complete your workout. If you are prone to run low on blood sugar, make sure to snack one to two hours before exercising. Make sure your snack or meal has proteins that will stable your blood sugar level and some fast-acting carbs. Make sure that you eat something with at least 20 grams of carbs and 20 grams of protein within two hours of completing your workout to replenish your glycogen stores, build-up your muscles and keep you energized.

Having such a snack will ensure that sugars are not reintroduced and that your body's metabolism keeps burning fat.

As you follow these tips, whatever intermittent fasting method you follow whether that's Warrior diet or alternating days, will cause your body to burn fat for your energy needs. This will shrink the size of your body's fat cells. It will reduce cellulite build-up in your butt and thighs and it will continue to improve your physique and health. Fast fat loss now becomes a reality within days of trying out intermittent fasting. This loss will become eminent when you measure the number of pounds you shed in just a few weeks.

Who should avoid the 5:2 Diet?

While the 5:2 intermittent fasting us relatively low risk, it is still important to see a doctor before attempting to fast if only to avoid unwanted risks. Women who are pregnant as well as those nursing a child should not consider fasting. The same is true with people afflicted by diabetes or hypoglycemia. In fact any illness that requires you avoid eating below a certain range of calories should make you think twice about fasting. Obese people suffering from heart problems and other organ issues should seek further advice from a doctor before considering intermittent fasting as a means of achieving weight loss and better health. People with adrenal fatigue or chronic stress should also avoid intermittent fasting.

Bonus Chapter – Avoid Binge Eating

An unwanted effect of intermittent fasting is binge eating. Binge eating usually occurs during the first few attempts at fasting where your cravings prompt you to "make up" for the missed food. It also occurs prior to fasting, where you feel conditioned to eat more in order to feel less hungry during the fast. The problem with this is it promptly restores your body's bad habits of relying on sugar for fuel, especially if you binge on snacks or sugar rich food. It reverses any metabolic changes and de-regulates your insulin, leptin and ghrelin levels. When this happens your body responds as if you came from a "starvation" experience and will start prompting you to eat and make up for lost weight.

To avoid binge eating, here are a few reminders and tips to keep in mind:

Plan your meals

Planning what to eat after a fasting session allows you to specify how many calories you will have and prevents the temptation of ordering everything on the menu. Even if you decide to eat out in order to break your fast, you should still make an effort to plan ahead. This will also ensure you have enough to pay for your meal as well too.

Avoid Sugar

In planning your meals, remember to avoid sugar-rich food. Sugar is a substance that throws off your metabolism and wreaks havoc on your insulin and leptin resistance. If you really want better health and a balanced weight, do what you can to avoid sugar at all costs. Your health is at stake.

Count Calories

Learn how much calories go into each serving of your food on feast days so that you know how much to reduce your food on fast days. This will keep you from guessing and prevent you from binging. It will also allow you to spread your meals in order to have maximum energy. The internet has so many calorie calculators and counters if you want to be specific.

Know what is Normal and Stick to It

The excuse of binge eaters would be that they didn't know they had exceeded the required calorie counts. You don't need a calorie counter and measure the calories of every meal. By establishing the servings you eat if each kind of food, you basically have an idea what normally fills you up and what exceeds it. Use that knowledge to guide how much you eat after every fast instead of your stomach's rumblings.

Organic Remedies for the Brain

It is true that as people get older, various functions of the body gradually decline. The muscles get weaker, the vision gets blurred, the ears get less sensitive to sound, and the blood vessels get less elastic over time, thus leading to various diseases that predispose the elderly to injuries. The same is true for the brain. Neurons die and the connections between these cells degenerate leading to gradual decline in cognition. With aging, there is impairment of short- and long-term memory, sensory and motor functions.

Though aging cannot be stopped from happening, its onset and progression can, however, be delayed. Well, aside from the anti-aging supplements and memory enhancers that you can buy from the market, there are still a lot of things that you can do to protect your brain from degenerative diseases, such as Alzheimer's and Parkinson's disease. Several studies have established the role of organic herbs and foods in keeping the brain healthy.

Here are some of the herbs that can enhance the functions of your hardworking brain:

1. Broccoli

Boost your brain power by eating a serving of broccoli every day. Just like Kale, broccoli belongs to the family of cruciferous vegetables which are known for their enormous antioxidant, vitamin, and mineral content. Broccoli contains a lot of compounds that have been shown to help delay the progression of degeneration of brain cells. One of them is lignan, which is a phytonutrient that has been known to act specifically on the brain. It boosts cognitive functions by improving one's learning capabilities, memory, and reasoning.

It is also rich in glucosinate, which is a compound that prevents the decrease in the levels of acetylcholine, a chemical mediator in several brain processes, such as movement and memory. A decrease in the levels of this neurotransmitter has been implicated in the development of Alzheimer's disease.

2. Avocado

Avocado had been in the dark for quite some time because of several misconceptions. It was initially believed to be unhealthy because of its high fat content. However, it was later on revealed that though they may be fatty, the types of fat it contains are not harmful at all. They were actually high density lipoproteins and omega- 3 fatty acids. Because of this, avocado has become the subject of researches that aim to study its beneficial effects.

Currently, avocado is known to contain a lot of nutrients, not only the fats mentioned above. It is rich in vitamin B complex (B1, B2, B3, B5, B6, B9, and B12), which is known to be neuroprotective, vitamin E, which is a potent scavenger for free radicals, and vitamins A, D, K and C, which all have beneficial effects not only to the brain but to other organs as well.

How does avocado protect the brain? First, the fat content of this fruit allows for good blood circulation in the brain. Omega-3 fatty acid has an anti-inflammatory property that protects the blood vessels from damage. Because HDLs facilitate the removal of cholesterol plaques from the lumen of the blood vessels, adequate blood flow to the various regions of the brain is achieved. This prevents stroke from occurring. Stroke is a consequence of decreased delivery of oxygen to the brain, which happens when there is occlusion of blood vessels.

Second, omega-3 fatty acids are associated with better mood. Studies found out that there is actually an inverse relationship between the levels of omega-3 fatty acids in the blood and the risk of depression and hostility. There is, on the other hand, a direct relationship between one's intelligence quotient (IQ) and omega-3 fatty acid levels.

And third, the vitamin K content of avocado protects the brain from hemorrhage. Vitamin K is needed in the activation of several clotting factors and deficiency of this vitamin can lead to excessive bleeding.

3. Coconut oil

Just like avocado, coconut oil has received a bad welcome from many health experts for the past few years because of its fat content. However, these speculations have been proven to be wrong. Coconut oil is trans-fat free. Trans-fat is a type of saturated fat that is known to cause several heart ailments. Unlike unsaturated fats, saturated fats solidify or precipitate under normal body temperature. Hence, they have a great tendency to form aggregates inside the blood vessels and cause obstruction.

Sticking to the walls of the vessel does not only cause obstruction of the flow of blood but it also stimulates the inflammatory process. In an attempt of the body to get rid of these sticky fats, the inflammatory cells and the platelets surround the plaque causing further harm. The more cells come into the site of obstruction, the more obstructed the vessel will become. Occlusion leads to decreased blood flow to the brain, which in turn leads to death of brain cells. With the death of these cells, the brain is less able to perform its functions.

Supplementation with coconut oil has also been found out to be very beneficial for people suffering from Alzheimer's type of dementia. Researchers claim that coconut oil can actually protect the brain cells from the damaging effects of a protein called beta-amyloid. These proteins are seen in patients with Alzheimer's disease as cellular deposits and have been implicated in the production of cognitive deficits typical of the said disease.

4. Spinach

As a child, you might have already appreciated the importance and health benefits of this herb as you watched Popeye the Sailorman's muscles get pumped up after dumping a canfull of spinach into his mouth. However, you might not have realized then that there is still a lot more to spinach than being a muscle-pumper.

Spinach is loaded with several micronutrients making it an all-in-one green leafy vegetable. It is packed with antioxidants making it a good anti-aging agent. It is also infused with multiple vitamins and minerals that make it an energy booster. Fiber is also etched in every corner of this vegetable. But the most important component of spinach that makes it a perfect brain food is folate or Vitamin B9.

Folic acid has long been used as a supplement by pregnant mothers as this can prevent the formation of spinal cord and brain abnormalities, called neural tube defects, in fetuses. These spinal and brain defects are commonly seen as masses of meninges and spinal cord herniating out of the skin of the back, usually in the lower portions. But the beneficial effects of folate are not only limited to fetuses and pregnant mothers, because everyone can benefit from its neuroprotective effects.

Folate promotes neural development, growth of new cells and formation of new connections among neurons. These connections are necessary for faster transmission of impulses to and from the brain. An increase in the level of this B vitamin is also associated with higher levels of neurotransmitters, most especially of dopamine and serotonin.

Dopamine is mainly responsible for motor functions, while serotonin is mainly responsible for the regulation of one's mood and sleep pattern. Serotonin is also the neurotransmitter that is implicated in sundown phenomenon, a disorder that is characterized by depressed mood during sunset and a manic or normal mood in the presence of sunlight. It was theorized that sunlight induces the production of serotonin leading to enhanced mood. Aside from spinach, folate can also be found in eggplant, celery and beans.

5. Olive Oil

Olive oil is not just great for cooking pastas, but it is also great in protecting your brain from age-related degeneration. Olive oil, just like avocado and coconut oil, is rich in polyunsaturated fats. Aside from preventing stroke, polyunsaturated fats promote the transmission of impulses to and from the nervous system. Fats facilitate myelination of nerves.

Normally, the brain transmits several signals within a second because of the presence of myelin sheath. This sheath does not only serve as protective covering of your nerves, but they also facilitate faster transmission of impulses. Without them, transmission will be disrupted and slower. An impulse normally travels through nerve A, then nerve B, then nerve C before it reaches its destination. However, if a person has deficient myelin, an impulse will not traverse its normal route. It can either go to nerve Z or to nerve A before it can reach its target cell. Olive oil also has a role in the regulation of one's mood.

Conclusion

So, are you convinced that the 5:2 Diet intermittent fasting method is the way to better health and weight loss? Or are you still thinking of trying out one of those new diets?

With a comparison of the differences of a diet from intermittent fasting as well as the differences between 5:2 and other methods, you should have by now a good grasp of what's in store for you. Except perhaps for a few people such as those with hypoglycemia, chronic stress, or are currently pregnant or nursing a baby, the 5:2 intermittent fasting method is much more applicable to anyone rather than LeanGains or the Warrior's Diet. It should be well within your capabilities to have a small meal twice a day or to work out while fasting.

The next step is to review the benefits, advantages, FAQ's and otherwise how to conduct intermittent fasting. If you feel the need for more information, look up Dr. Mosley's blog or his book. Otherwise, you can start by mapping out what a normal meal is like and what would a fasting meal size be. Then if you still want proper guidance, try out a 12 hour fast and see how well your body responds. If in doubt, consult your doctor and ask about any risks or symptoms that you need to be wary. Check for any risks to your health such as chronic stress, diabetes, or hypoglycemia. Then make the necessary changes and revisit your doctor for additional counsel and permission.

Once you're ready, try out your first day of intermittent fasting and see how your body reacts to it. Just remember to watch out for binge eating and be consistent when you eat so that your body can reprogram itself and adapt to your new lifestyle.

Better health and weight loss are just around the corner as you settle into your new lifestyle and start discovering the benefits of the 5:2 Diet.

One Last Thing...

If you enjoyed this book or found it useful I'd be very grateful if you'd post a short review on Amazon. Your support really does make a difference and I read all the reviews personally so I can get your feedback and make this book even better.

If you'd like to leave a review then all you need to do is click the review link on this book's page...

Thank You so Much

www.ingramcontent.com/pod-product-compliance
Lightning Source LLC
Chambersburg PA
CBHW071352310526
45790CB00018B/1425